# The **YOGA** of
# GHOST HUNTING

# The **YOGA** of GHOST HUNTING

*Tips and Techniques
for Psychic Protection and More*

**Richard Salva**
Author of
*The Reincarnation of Abraham Lincoln*

crystal clarity **publishers**
nevada city; california

**Crystal Clarity Publishers**
Nevada City, CA 95959

Copyright © 2010 by Richard Salva
Originally published in 2010 by Crystar Press
Published 2014

ISBN: 978-1-56589-288-0
ePub: 978-1-56589-506-5
Printed in the United States of America

*Cover design: Tejindra Scott Tully*
*Cover photograph of woods by Antonio Romei*

Library of Congress Cataloging-in-Publication Data

Salva, Richard.
The Yoga of Ghost Hunting : tips and techniques for psychic
protection and more / Richard Salva. — 1st ed.
p. cm.
ISBN 978-1-56589-288-0 (tradepaper, bw images)
—ISBN 978-1-56589-506-5
1. Ghosts. 2. Ghosts—Research--Methodology. 3. Yoga. 4.
Yogananda, Paramhansa, 1893-1952. I. Title.

BF1461.S325 2014
133.1—dc22
2011013512

www.crystalclarity.com
800.424.1055 or 530.478.7600
clarity@crystalclarity.com

**06 14**

TO MY WIFE LAURA,
WHO BRAVED THE UNKNOWN WITH ME

# ACKNOWLEDGMENTS

I would like to thank the following people who contributed to the development of this book:

Sandie La Nae

Janice Oberding

Laura Salva

Bill (our helpful ghost transitioner)

Raghu Clark

Matthew O. Sloan

Gurudas Barrett

Tejindra Scott Tully

David Jensen

Swami Kriyananda

   and Crystal Clarity Publishers

# CONTENTS

# ILLUSTRATIONS

# INTRODUCTION

As a daily practitioner for more than thirty years of meditation and the deeper teachings of yoga, I have found it curious that, even though I have not sought them out, I have crossed paths with ghosts and other astral forces.

In fact, when I was asked to lecture on my book *The Reincarnation of Abraham Lincoln*\* at a paranormal conference a few years ago, I realized that I had a lot to say on the subjects of ghosts and ghost hunting.

It also became clear as I spoke that most of what I was saying was new to my listeners. I was presenting a view of ghost hunting that veteran ghost hunters had never heard before.

In addition, I was aware of techniques and concepts that could help ghost hunters achieve greater success in their efforts and avoid some of the pitfalls of their pastime.

Here, then, is the essence of what I have shared at ghost hunting conferences, along with additional helpful tips and techniques, all based on ancient yogic teachings.

\* Published by Crystal Clarity Publishers.

People go ghost hunting for a variety of reasons. Ghost hunts can be fun and fascinating, yet there is much more to them than that. Serious visitors to haunted houses recognize that what they are doing may bring answers to some of life's Big Questions—Is there life after death? Are ghosts the spirits of people who have died? Is it possible to find proof of these subtle realities?

Once we know more about what ghosts are and the world in which they live, we can gain a better understanding of what we may experience on a ghost hunt.

As I said, the information I am sharing here is based on the deeper teachings of yoga as taught by great spiritual masters and world teachers.

If you look at the front cover of the Beatles' *Sergeant Pepper* album, you will see near the top right-hand corner a man with long dark hair and bright eyes. This is Paramhansa Yogananda, author of the spiritual classic *Autobiography of a Yogi.**

Yogananda's powerful bestselling book has inspired millions throughout the world, including such well-known individuals as the Beatles and Elvis Presley. In one of the later chapters of Yogananda's autobiography, he relates an amazing experience—three months after the passing of his Guru, Swami Sri Yukteswar, the great spiri-

* The 1946 original unedited edition, pictured on the next page, is published by Crystal Clarity Publishers. All quotations in this book from *Autobiography of a Yogi* are from the Crystal Clarity edition.

tual master physically resurrected himself (raised himself from the dead). He embraced Yogananda and shared deep teachings. In that chapter, the just-materialized Sri Yukteswar told Yogananda many fascinating details about the afterlife and the energy sphere that ghosts inhabit, which he called the "astral universe."

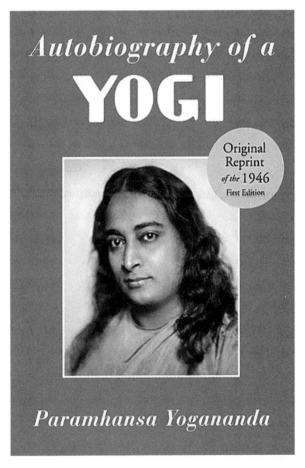

**Autobiography of a Yogi front cover.**

# Chapter One

## Just Where Are Ghosts Coming From?

Sri Yukteswar told Yogananda that "[t] here are many astral planets, teeming with astral beings. The inhabitants use astral planes, or masses of light, to travel from one planet to another."

"The astral world," he explained, "is infinitely beautiful, clean, pure, and orderly."

"Various spheric mansions or vibratory regions are provided for good and evil spirits. Good ones can travel freely, but the evil spirits are confined to limited zones."*

In this fascinating chapter in Yogananda's autobiography, Sri Yukteswar describes what astral beings look like, what their bodies are made of (prana, or "lifetrons"), what they eat, what people look like when they arrive in the astral world after death, how astral beings communicate, and more.

* *Autobiography of a Yogi*, p. 402.

"The ordinary astral universe," he said, "is peopled with millions of astral beings who have come, more or less recently, from the earth." In addition, he went on, there are also non-human beings, which he described as "fairies, mermaids, fishes, animals, goblins, gnomes, demigods and spirits."*

Sri Yukteswar also spoke of the great size of the astral universe.

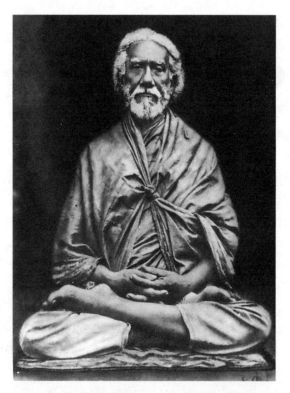

**Swami Sri Yukteswar, incarnation of wisdom, guru of Yogananda**

* *Autobiography of a Yogi*, p. 402.

We know that the physical universe is unbelievably vast. Scientists have clocked the speed of light at 186,000 miles a second. Going at that speed and traveling from earth, it would take a spaceship more than four years to reach the nearest star.

Keeping that in mind, consider that there are approximately one hundred billion stars in our galaxy. And there are about one hundred billion galaxies in the physical universe. Between most galaxies are wide reaches of space.

So, what we can see through our telescopes is pretty big. But the astral universe is much bigger.

To give an idea of the size difference between the two, Sri Yukteswar said that the physical universe is like the basket that hangs under the huge hot air balloon of the astral plane.*

This analogy is inexact in that the physical universe is not *suspended from* the astral universe in any physical way. Rather, part of the subtle astral universe *merges with* the smaller physical universe—lying behind it, so to speak. The separation between the two universes is caused by the vibrational difference between matter and pure energy.

Throughout this book we will explore some of the ways in which Sri Yukteswar's description of the astral world relates to ghosts and ghost hunting.

* *Autobiography of a Yogi,* p. 402.

Astral Universe
(balloon)

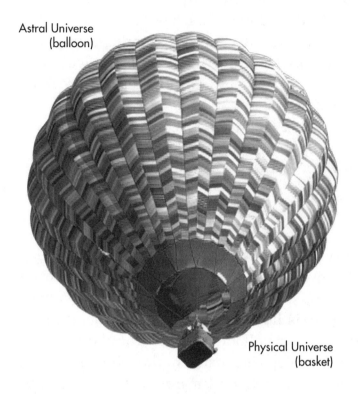

Physical Universe
(basket)

**Relative sizes of astral and physical universes,
as per Sri Yukteswar's hot air balloon analogy**
(Original Image: FreeDigitalPhotos.net)

## Chapter Two

## A SPIRITUAL BENEFIT OF GHOST HUNTING

I know. Most people probably aren't thinking about spiritual benefits while engaged in a ghost hunt. But the fact remains that an essential aspect of these activities can lead to spiritual growth.

Why are ghost hunts exciting? Because ghosts are scary. And why are they scary? Well, for a number of reasons; but to a large degree, because ghosts are invisible.

Think about it. What is a ghost? Something you can't see that can touch you, influence you, physically chill you, even speak to you.

Man fears the unknown.

Whatever our reason for going on a ghost hunt, or the exact cause of our interest and excitement, we cannot deny that fear is part of the equation.

And this brings us back to that spiritual benefit we were discussing.

Fear is an obstacle to spiritual growth. If you are afraid of anything, in that area at least, your inner growth is blocked.

How do we overcome fear?

Sri Yukteswar gave this advice: "Look fear in the face," he said, "and it will cease to trouble you."

And that is exactly what people do on ghost hunts. They seek out what they are afraid of and face their fears.

When Sri Yukteswar was young he went on a ghost hunt; in fact, he told Yogananda the story of his ghost hunt to illustrate the principle of "looking fear in the face."

He said, "My mother once tried to frighten me with [a] story of a ghost in a dark chamber. I went there immediately, and expressed my disappointment at having missed the ghost. Mother never told me another horror-tale."*

Sri Yukteswar's story, though brief and amusing, hints at his self-mastery, evident to everyone who met him. But he wasn't the only spiritually advanced soul to face and overcome the fear of death. Yogis in India sometimes meditate in burial grounds.† Christian monks in medieval times

---

* *Autobiography of a Yogi*, p. 105.

† Yogananda himself, as a high school student in India, observed this practice. As he wrote on p. 83 of his autobiography: "The passing months found me less frequently in the classroom than in secluded spots along the Calcutta bathing ghats. The adjoining crematory grounds, especially gruesome at night, are considered highly attractive by the yogi. He who would find the Deathless Essence must not be dismayed by a few unadorned skulls. Human

used the skulls of their deceased brothers as drinking bowls. The meditations of the Buddha and St. Antony of the Desert were disturbed by rowdy phantoms, trying to frighten them away from their spiritual practices.

These great souls faced their fears and overcame them. And so can you.

---

inadequacy becomes clear in the gloomy abode of miscellaneous bones. My midnight vigils were thus of a different nature from the scholors." Later on that same page he added, "Braving the ghouls, I was exhuming a knowledge not found in lecture halls."

# Tips and Techniques

The next time you go on a ghost hunt, don't just allow yourself to get swept into the group atmosphere and the thrill of the occasion.

Every so often, take a few moments to introspect. How are you reacting to your experience? Are you afraid? If so, why?

Honestly look at whatever is scaring you and mentally face it head on. You might try visualizing for a few moments your worst fear coming true, and mentally accept it. Once you've mastered your fear, at least to some extent, carry on with the ghost hunt. But continue to keep a watch on your feelings. Little by little, work to strengthen your courage and sense of fearlessness.

Affirm mentally, "I live in the fortress of my higher Self. As long as I remain in the heart of it, nothing and no one can harm me."

If you continue with this practice, over time you will find yourself less frightened of the disembodied. More importantly, you will be less fearful of many formerly scary aspects of your life.

# Chapter Three

## HOW TO CLEAR YOUR AURA

Recently, after presenting a lecture at a paranormal conference, the conference leader asked me about spirit possession. She said that occasionally people have felt after a ghost hunt that they brought spirits home with them. Can this really happen, and if so, what can be done about it?

In response, I shared with her some of Yogananda's teachings on this subject.

Yogananda pointed out that sometimes when people get very drunk, they black out and find themselves hours later in a strange location with no recollection of what they did in the meantime or how they got there.

Similarly, Yogananda cautioned against allowing our minds to become "blank" during meditation (or indeed, at any other time). He gave the analogy of leaving a car running with the door open. Any "tramp spirit" wandering by could hi-jack the vehicle.

There is a code of conduct in the astral world. No highly evolved soul would ever enter and use another's body or interfere with their lives.

However, a lower astral being wouldn't think twice about it.

Many years ago I went through a period of emotional vulnerability. After a few months, I sensed that a disembodied spirit had invaded my energy field, or aura.

When our auras are weak, they leave openings through which other spirits can enter. In such cases, their energy fields will overlap with ours. When that happens, those who see astral beings might glimpse astral faces peeking over our shoulders or otherwise hanging out in our auras.

What are the effects of such minor spirit possession? And how can we know that a ghost has attached himself to us?

When you are in such a state you will experience a lack of inner clarity and a feeling of uncleanness, as if the water of your life had become polluted. Thoughts that are not your own, that have nothing to do with your life, may run through your mind. Similarly, you may feel emotions that are disconnected from your experiences, or a strong overreaction to those experiences.

A ghost may attach himself to you during a period of emotional turmoil because he feels a connection with your state of mind. He may harbor the hope that he can work out his own desires or karma through you. In that case, he will try to influence your reactions to things, to pull on your thoughts or emotions so that you will act as he would in your situation.

This is, of course, an unhealthy state. If you are experiencing anything like this, you will want to free yourself as soon as possible.

When I briefly had an experience of this type, I drew on Yogananda's teachings and techniques for clearing the aura—described below and in other chapters—and removed that spirit's energy field from mine.

# Tips and Techniques

***The Importance of Centering Yourself:*** By sending an electrical current through a wire, you can magnetize the wire and create a magnetic field around it. Interrupting the electrical flow would weaken the magnetic field or make it disappear altogether.

Similarly, a subtle energy channel runs through the center of your physical body, in the deep spine. When the energy in that channel flows freely, the "electrical field" of your aura is bright and strong. Anything that interrupts that energy flow weakens your aura.

And a weak aura is an open invitation to a ghost to enter your psychic space.

During ghost hunts (and all the time, as much as you can), while sitting or standing, try to keep your spine straight with your body as relaxed as possible.

***Centering Exercise 1:*** Stand upright with your feet flat on the floor, your weight slightly forward on the balls of your feet.

Close your eyes and visualize a straight line running through the center of your body. This line extends down into the floor, and up through the top of the head into the ceiling above.

Now, relax your body into alignment with that line. Keep in mind that a straight spine is the natural position for your body. Hold just enough tension in your muscles to maintain this erect posture. Don't be stiff, but remain as relaxed as possible with your spine straight.

(There is a certain amount of natural curvature to the spine. However, visualizing a straight line running through the center of your spine will help ensure that only the correct and healthy amount of curvature is coming into play at any given moment.)

***Centering Exercise 2:*** At the end of the previous exercise, and keeping your eyes closed, sway your body slightly to the left and right. When you sway to the left, resist that movement mentally by imagining your body swaying right—and vice versa.

This exercise will help you center your consciousness in the deep spine.

After you have practiced for a time, stop swaying and relax, standing upright with eyes closed, enjoying your deepened awareness.

***Aura Strengthening/Clearing 1:*** Our hands are like magnets. We can send a great deal of energy through them, which is why some healers use the technique of "laying on hands."

The human aura is like a cocoon of energy and light that surrounds our physical bodies. Here is

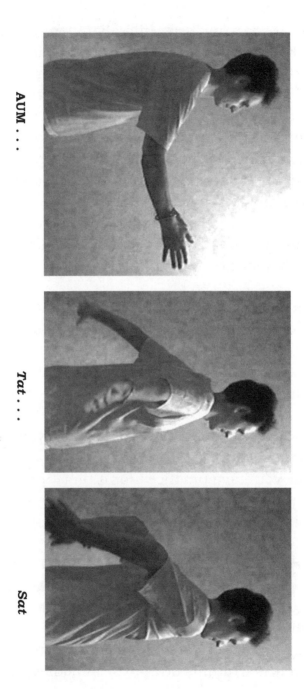

AUM . . .    Tat . . .    Sat

how you can strengthen your aura with the powerful energy flowing through your hands.

A. Standing upright, rub the palms of your hands together. Feel the heat and energy generated in the palms of the hands.

B. Now, fully extend your arms in front of you, keeping the palms of your hands together.

C. Next, turn your hands so that your palms are facing away from each other, and simultaneously swing your arms around your body until your palms are touching behind you.

D. Then, swing your arms forward again, ascribing a circle around your body, until your palms are touching in front of you once more.

E. Continue to swing your arms forward and backward, slowly and consciously, over and over. With each movement, strengthen your aura—sending energy through your hands and into your aura by the direct application of your will.

 Your hands are touching the outside of your aura. Feel your aura growing stronger with each movement, with each pass of your hands.

F. Now, we will add one more element to your practice.

 • When your hands are in front of you, chant aloud the sacred word AUM (pronounced "OM").

- While your hands are swinging around you, going toward your back, chant TAT (rhymes with "hot").
- When they have completed the circle and are touching behind you, chant SAT (also rhymes with "hot").

("AUM TAT SAT" is an ancient Sanskrit mantra of great power. Chanting it aligns you with the highest light and spirit within you. It is an effective and powerful instrument for strengthening your aura.)

When you have mastered all the elements of this technique, practice it with your eyes closed. Consciously feel the energy you are pouring into your aura through your hands and your will.

Use this technique whenever your aura is weak and you feel vulnerable to negative psychic influences.

Below are photos of myself practicing this technique.

I've also posted an online video of myself practicing AUM TAT SAT.

*http://www.youtube.com/watch?v=gCBZxAjqwP0*

**Aura Strengthening/Clearing 2:** Our minds are very powerful. Whatever you strongly and consistently believe about yourself will, in some manner or form, come to pass.

The world is like an interactive movie. We can influence it through our thoughts and mental images.

This is why positive affirmations and visualizations are so important.

We can use the power of the mind to strengthen our auras.

Sit on the floor in a cross-legged meditative pose, or in a chair with the spine straight and away from the back of the chair, your feet flat on the floor, and your hands placed at the juncture of the thighs and abdomen with the palms turned upward.

Visualize a coccoon of light all around your body, extending several feet above the top of your head and down around you on all sides until it ends below your feet.

See this cocoon as strong and bright with light. Just as you can use a dial switch to turn up a light, use your will to brighten your aura until it is brilliant, shining, and radiant.

Lastly, imagine that this cocoon of light has a Teflon coating. Whatever touches it cannot stick to it, but will easily slide off and away from you.

Use this visualization before and during ghost hunts, as needed.

### Aura Strengthening/Clearing 3:

Above, I mentioned the "AUM *Tat Sat*" mantra.

There is another very powerful and ancient Sanskrit mantra which, when repeated with deep concentration, can clear your aura of foreign influences.

It is called the *Mahamrityanjaya* mantra and the words are as follows:

> *AUM, triambakam yajaamahe sugandim,*
> *pushti-vaardhanam*
> *Urvaarukameva bhandanaan mrityor*
> *mokshiya Maamritaat, AUM.*

### *Translation:*

We worship the three-eyed One (the divine Spirit whose spiritual eye is open) who is fragrant (with joy and life) and who nourishes all beings.

May He liberate us from death and bring us immortality, even as the cucumber is severed from its bondage to the creeper.

This mantra may take some time to memorize, but it is worth the effort.

Seated in a meditative posture with your eyes closed, repeat the mantra aloud at least thrice. At the same time, visualize any ties to astral beings as if they were twigs and branches connected to your aura. See in your mind's eye that you are holding a sword of spiritual power. Mentally wield this sword to cut away those negative connections. Then, cast those branch-like connections into a blazing fire.

You could also repeat this mantra while seated before an actual fire, and throw rice seeds (symbolizing negative connections or attachments) into the flames with the chanting of the final AUM at the end of each repetition.

Practice this technique until you feel all outside influences disappear.

If you would like help learning it, Crystal Clarity Publishers sells a CD or MP3 recording of Swami Kriyananda chanting the *Mahamrityunjaya* mantra. I highly recommend this recording.

Or you can purchase this mantra individually for download from iTunes™. Search for "Mahamrityunjaya Chant" chanted by Swami Kriyananda.

Visit: http://crystalclarity.com/product.php?code=MM

I have also posted a Youtube video of myself chanting the mantra several times.

Go to: www.youtube.com watch?v=z6Hp5WGnhRM

### A Note about Benign Spirits:

We've been discussing lower astral entities who would cavalierly take over your body and mind in order to selfishly work out their own karma and desires. But higher spirits also populate the astral sphere, and these spirits can serve as a positive influence. They, too, might touch our auras, but only very gently and in blessing.

When I began writing *The Reincarnation of Abraham Lincoln*, I went to a shaman in Tahoe, California for a psychic reading. At about the time when the reading was supposed to begin, she came out of her office to tell me she was running late. Before speaking to me, she looked over my shoulder and smiled. I wondered what that was about but said nothing at the time.

During the reading with the shaman, we discussed a number of things. At one point I mentioned my Lincoln book. She beamed and told me that, when she had come out to speak to me before the reading, she had seen Abraham Lincoln in my aura. She knew I was going to bring him up in our conversation.

I found what she said to be deeply meaningful.

While working on *The Reincarnation of Abraham Lincoln* I tried to tune into Lincoln's spirit—and I often felt that I succeeded, sensing his presence, encouragement, and guidance. The shaman's words validated my experience.

To connect with an evolved being mentally, psychically, or spiritually, is always beneficial. Their sole purpose is to bless and inspire, not to control or interfere with one's own natural, spiritual evolution. Their only desire is your best welfare.

# Chapter Four

## A QUICK WORD ABOUT COLORS

We've dealt so far with certain aspects of psychic protection, but there is a minor one we haven't touched on.

It's fashionable among those who go ghost hunting to wear black, like the darkness from which ghostly experiences come. Black also symbolizes the unknown.

However, from the standpoint of psychic self-protection, black is the worst color to wear.

Black clothing attracts darkness and negativity. Among the various kinds of ghost hunting experiences you can have, the most unpleasant ones can be drawn to you, at least partly, through wearing black.

In that case, what color should you wear if you like to go ghost hunting but want to draw more of a fun experience?

# Tips and Techniques

From a yogic perspective, the various colors represent the spectrum of life's experience and various levels of consciousness.

Every color has its positive and negative aspects. For example, a bright or rich green (like a sward of grass in springtime, or slightly darker as in a deep forest) can suggest health and prosperity, while a sickly green implies jealousy or decay. Generally speaking, brighter and clearer tones represent higher states of consciousness and darker and muddier tones represent something undesirable and unhealthy.

From a psychic-protection point of view, the lighter and more joyful the garb you wear, the better.

Have fun with the colors you wear on a ghost hunt! If the purpose is to entertain yourself, why not let your clothes add to the experience?

If white is too bright for you or others in the group, try yellow or orange or blue or gold or turquoise, or . . . whatever invigorates you.

The general rule of thumb is: Choose colors that lift and strengthen your spirit, rather than the opposite.

# Chapter Five

## TYPES OF GHOSTS

If you've been ghost hunting for any length of time, you've probably observed that there are different kinds of ghosts and levels of ghostly experiences.

Just as there are various personality types among the residents of any apartment building, some ghosts are grouchy, others are in a relatively good mood; some are noisy, while some are peaceful and unobtrusive; some are friendly, others not so much.

In my own otherworldly forays, I've experienced everything from a pure and joyful light it was a pleasure to encounter to a dark energy that made my skin crawl.

Earlier, we quoted Sri Yukteswar speaking about higher and lower planes in the astral universe. There are stories of spirits from the higher astral planes acting as instruments of light in this world—like the ghosts who visited Scrooge in Charles Dickens' *A Christmas Carol.*

Here's a fascinating example of what I mean: in the middle of a Pacific aerial battle during WW II, a pilot was helped by a ghost. The windshield of his airplane had shattered under a hail of bullets, leaving the pilot's eyes damaged and his face all bloody. The pilot couldn't see; he was literally flying blind.

Suddenly, his radio came to life with the voice of a pilot apparently from another squadron. This helpful pilot carefully and lovingly guided the blind aviator to a safe landing on an aircraft carrier. When the rescued pilot spoke to those who helped him out of his airplane, he was surprised to hear that they had seen no sign of his savior's airplane. He was even more astonished when he learned that the name his "wingman" had given him was that of a pilot who had died earlier in the war.*

Similarly, Paramhansa Yogananda's spirit appeared to a man who lived under the Iron Curtain, saving him from imprisonment and worse.

Yogananda's disciple, Swami Kriyananda, described the incident in his book, *The New Path*:

"In 1955 I went to Switzerland. . . . There I met a lady from Czechoslovakia who told me a story

---

* I read this fascinating story years ago in an old paperback of ghost stories in wartime. Unfortunately, I cannot remember the title or the author, nor have I been able to locate the book online.

concerning Professor Novicky, the late leader of a small [meditation] group in Prague.

"'One day,' she said, 'after Yogananda's passing, a stranger came to Professor Novicky and requested instruction in yoga. The professor didn't know what to do. Normally he kept his spiritual activities a secret so as not to expose himself to persecution. If this man was a genuine seeker, the professor would want to help him. But if he was a communist government spy, any admission of interest in yoga might result in a prison sentence for him. Our friend prayed for guidance. Suddenly, standing behind that self-proclaimed 'devotee,' Paramhansa Yogananda appeared. Slowly the Master shook his head, then vanished. Professor Novicky told the man he had come to the wrong place for information. Sometime later, he learned that the man was indeed a government spy.

"'I am free to tell this story now,' my informant continued, 'for the good professor died recently, of natural causes.'"*

_____

* *The New Path*, p. 258.

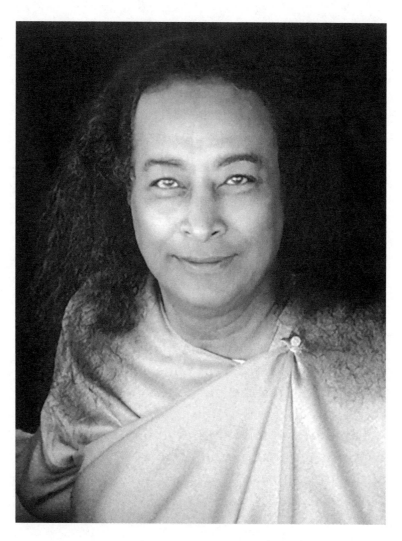

**Paramhansa Yogananda**

# Tips and Techniques

Many deceased folks who are spiritually advanced are open to helping people. We can tune into their spirits by focusing mentally on an individual soul, as Professor Novicky did with Paramhansa Yogananda.

As Sri Yukteswar said, higher spirits are freer than lower ones. They have more power; light banishes darkness.

Everyone is blessed by an individual who acts as a direct instrument of light for them. It could be a great soul like Christ or Buddha, or someone less obviously spiritual or well known, like the deceased pilot mentioned above.

Choose a spiritual guide with whom you feel in tune. (If no one comes to mind, feel free to call on Yogananda, who is a very powerful and open channel of Light.) Place that person's picture on a small table, perhaps with a lit candle, creating a little altar of sorts. Sit and look at the picture for a while. Then, close your eyes and meditate. Send a mental message to that individual from the spiritual eye at the point between the eyebrows. Listen for and feel his or her response in your heart.

In time you will create a strong bond of light between yourself and your spiritual guide.

Deepening your connection with your guide can be very useful if you run into a ghost deeply stuck in darkness. Often, just one thought of your guide can free you from danger and fear.

# Chapter Six

## IS IT A GHOST OR SOMETHING ELSE?

A t the end of the last chapter, I mentioned how a ghost can become stuck in darkness. Because of some terrible life experience—personal betrayal, grievous loss, guilt over a mistake, or for a similar reason—he was thrown into a profoundly negative state of mind from which he hasn't yet escaped.

Yogananda made an interesting statement in *Autobiography of a Yogi*. He wrote that "thoughts are universally and not individually rooted."*

What he meant was—no matter where we are and at any time, we can tune into *any* state of consciousness. The entire broadband of thought that mankind has accessed is always at our "fingertips," waiting for us to dial in our mental radios. We are always free to tune into the "radio stations" of geniuses, or villains, or saints, or

* *Autobiography of a Yogi*, p. 154.

failures. It's up to us—and our mental habits, which can be changed.

When we really like a radio station for its music or talk show, what do we do? We carefully spin the tuning dial until it is centered on that wavelength, then we crank up the volume.

We do the same thing mentally, whenever we are happy or sad—focusing on a positive or negative thought until it fills our consciousness. Then we increase the volume by feeding in our emotions.

And this is essentially the same thing that ghosts do, except they've been doing it for a longer period of time. They focus on a particular negative image or thought, creating a feedback loop between that image and the emotions it evokes.

Imagine a ghost inhabiting a building for hundreds of years. The longer he's been stuck there, the more energy he's channeled into his negative feedback loop, and the stronger the mental/emotional habit he's created for himself. Simultaneously, he's created an atmosphere in his building that makes it easier for you or me to access similar thoughts and feelings there.

It's as if someone were playing a rap song from a boom box in that place; it would take a concerted act of will to ignore it and not to walk in step to its beat.

But there is yet something else that can happen in these situations.

Sometimes, a ghost's mental/emotional feedback loop can draw non-ghostly entities to that location.

Whenever someone focuses one-pointedly on a thought or feeling, they can attract a spirit deeply in tune with that thought or feeling. (In India they call higher spirits of this type *devas*.)

For example, on a positive level, if you were to concentrate deeply on non-violence, seeking to manifest harmlessness in thought, word, and action—returning love for hatred, and so on—you may be visited in meditation by the spirit of Mahatma Gandhi or Jesus Christ. (Marvelous experiences like these have happened to many people.)

Conversely, if a man were to obsess on jealousy, he would not only open a psychic doorway for other people around him to experience that emotion—in time he could attract a spirit who has dived so deeply into jealousy that he has become a virtual embodiment of it.

This is the reason why some people visiting houses where truly horrible things have taken place have experienced not only ghosts, but other, very dark and scary manifestations: black clouds, poltergeist activities intended to scare or injure, and so on.

Of course, I highly recommend if you find your-self confronted by such a dark and dangerous entity to leave that location as quickly as you can. Little good can come from exposing oneself to such toxic energies.

# Tips and Techniques

*For Mental Clarity:* The best way to clear your mind is to keep your attention fixed at the point midway between the eyebrows, or spiritual eye. This is the seat of will power and concentration in the physical body. If your mind is strongly centered at the spiritual eye, it is very difficult for any person or spirit to interfere with your thought processes.

The forehead is the home of the frontal lobe—the most advanced part of the brain. Yogis who have calmly and firmly held their minds at this point have perfected their ability to concentrate and have accessed very high and deep states of consciousness.

When on a ghost hunt, if you feel a deceased soul's sadness (or another negative emotion) overwhelming you, bring your mind to the spiritual eye. Like Harry Potter when faced with a "dementor," focus on a positive thought until it fills your mind. Remember, though it seems unlikely in a negatively charged atmosphere, positive thoughts are just as available to you. All you have to do is adjust your mental radio dial.

In fact, I would recommend memorizing a positive affirmation—such as "I am joyful, every free;

I am free in the Light"—before you go on a ghost hunt.

With practice, you will discover an inner freedom unknown to you. No matter what situation you find yourself in—the ambiance of the room you're in, or the attitude of the group you're with—*your* mental radio broadcast can remain serene and light.

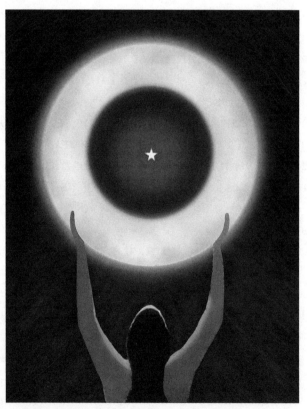

**In meditation, the spiritual eye looks like this.**
(Painting by Swami Kriyananda)

# Chapter Seven

## HOW TO BANISH SPIRITS

M any years ago I worked on the staff of a summer yoga program at Ananda Village in Nevada City, California. I had various duties, but one day an unusual task was added to my list.

An expectant mother in the program was having difficulties. She was sleeping at night in her van, the back of which had been converted into a makeshift camper. The van was parked in the midst of a small mountain glade.

Several times she had woken in the middle of the night, hearing the sounds of movement outside her van. Afterward the van would begin rocking, almost violently. At the same time, the child in her womb started kicking—"Going crazy," as she put it. In the midst of all this turmoil, the woman saw no movement or shapes when she pulled aside the shades and peered out her window. Apparently, there was nothing there.

Naturally, the woman was frightened by these experiences. She came to me for help. I offered to trade sleeping quarters until the problem was solved. That night the woman stayed indoors while I carried my sleeping bag up the hill and settled myself in her tent, located next to where she usually parked her van.

Before going to bed I sat upright in meditation and sent out positive energy, doing my best to fill the small mountain glade with light. If the entity was a disturbed human spirit, I wished him or her well. If it was something else, some kind of malevolent being, I willed it gone from that place.

After a time, I lay down and fell asleep.

At one point, hours later in the middle of the night, I woke up suddenly. Listening intently, I heard no sounds around the tent, but I felt a presence out there.

Sitting up in meditation, once again I sent energy and light out to that area. Simultaneously blessing the surroundings and anyone or anything that needed healing, and banishing any darkness, I raised my hands and chanted AUM many times.

Before long I felt a deep peace settle over the surrounding area, and I went back to sleep.

The next morning I described to the woman my experiences and what I had done. That night, she returned to the glade and her van. From then on she had no more problems with hostile spirits.

# Tips and Techniques

**Remember:** No darkness can harm you if you are acting as an instrument of the Light. The more you act as such an instrument, the stronger in light you will become.

Just as a tougher arm wrestler will defeat a weaker opponent, in an encounter between darkness and light the stronger force will always win out.

The amount of light our little egos can generate is limited. To channel a greater light, we have to get ourselves out of the picture. While sending light into that glade, I wasn't thinking about myself. Rather, I had forgotten myself in serving a greater cause. I wasn't depending on my own strength, but instead asked inwardly to act as an instrument of a greater light—specifically the light that shone through my great Guru, Paramhansa Yogananda.

That light was clearly greater than whatever darkness had been attracted to that glade, as it swiftly banished the entity or brought peace to that troubled spirit.

You, too, can act as an instrument of light. Start practicing now by mentally sending light to those you know who are in need. Concentrate on your spiritual guide—the greatest source of light with whom you feel a connection. Mentally ask your spiritual guide to help you become a channel of that same light.

Then, rub your hands together until you feel the energy in the palms. Raise your hands and, chanting AUM, send that light out into the world.

Important: Don't try, right at the start, to banish very strong or deeply entrenched darkness. Wait until you have become a strong channel of light. If you are unsure whether you are ready, leave it be until you *are* sure. Start small and focus on building your "light muscles." If you keep at it, you will become a powerful instrument of light and no dark or meddlesome spirit will trouble you.

# Chapter Eight

## *You* ARE A GHOST

If you were to view your hand through an electron microscope, you would see tiny particles of matter spinning around each other. Our bodies are composed mostly of space. Remove the space from your body and condense all the little particles together and you would have a block of mass so small you couldn't even see it.

Your body is a holding pattern of energy, an illusion of matter.

Our physical bodies are ghosts.

Do you believe that your physical body is who and what you are? (This is the premise, after all, for our first question about ghosts: Do we die when our physical bodies die?)

The essence of our belief that we are our physical forms stems partly from our daily, moment-by-moment experience of the sense inputs of touch, smell, taste, sight, and hearing. It also arises from our modern psychological dependence on physical science, which measures everything by mass, weight, and motion.

Almost certainly most of us assume our bodies *are* us, and make decisions based on that premise. Our physical bodies, and the physical world around us, are quite compelling. Our sense of touch seems so real—we don't stop to think that the sensations we are feeling are electrical impulses coursing through our nervous systems and interpreted by our brains.

Scientists tell us that the molecules in our bodies change every seven years. Our physical bodies have no lasting reality. And yet, you and I continue on.

*Who* are you? *What* are you? If not a physical body, what about your personality?

Most of us would say, if asked, that if our physical forms do not define us, then certainly our personalities do; ergo, the study of psychology.

And yet our personalities, the ways in which we express ourselves, shift as we pass through childhood, adolescence, adulthood, and old age. If we go through a devastating experience, our personalities could change dramatically. The same is true, in an opposite way, if we experience some type of spiritual conversion.

Well, you respond, my body and personality may shift through life, but I'm still ME.

You're absolutely right. But who is the "ME" you are referring to?

Who or what are you, if not a body or a personality?

A yogi would answer that you are a spirit, temporarily inhabiting a physical body, temporarily manifesting a particular personality.

In my book *The Reincarnation of Abraham Lincoln*, I explain that we put on a physical body when we reincarnate, like a suit or jacket that we wear for awhile, until it becomes un-wearable and we shrug it off, only to put on a new "physical suit" years later. (The same thing is true, to a large degree, with our personalities.)

People who lose a limb say they can still feel the limb there, although physically it is gone. Kirlian photographs have been taken of leaves after a part of them was snipped off. In each case, the energy aura of the entire leaf, whole and intact, remained.

There is, apparently, an energy body that lies behind the physical body.

We are not "bodies that have souls." We are "souls that have bodies." Our spirits are our lasting reality. They are the "ME" we refer to when we talk about that part of us that never changes.

A great woman saint from India, Ananda Moyi Ma, told Paramhansa Yogananda, "My consciousness has never associated itself with this temporary body. Before I came on this earth, Father, 'I was the same.' As a little girl, 'I was the same.' I grew into womanhood, but still 'I was the same.'. . . And, Father, in front of you now, 'I am the same.' Ever afterward, though the dance of creation change around me in the hall of eternity, 'I shall be the same.'"*

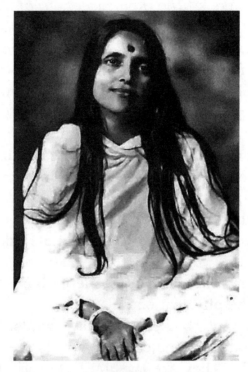

**Ananda Moyi Ma**

On the deepest level, what Anandamoyi Ma said is true for you and me and everyone.

Little more than a hundred years from now, all of us will be gone from this world. Little that we

* *Autobiography of a Yogi*, p. 440.

say and do and experience will be remembered. This planet—itself a big ghost that is constantly changing and has no lasting reality—will have other people "adorning it" (as Sri Yukteswar humorously put it), living their lives, learning their lessons, all briefly hypnotized by the 3D and sensory-integrated movie of physical existence.

Ghosts are like us, except that one layer of unreality has been removed: their physical bodies. And we are like them, except that for a brief period of time we are using our physical bodies to play our roles on the stage of the physical world.

Paramhansa Yogananda pointed out that we all turn into ghosts at night. In our dreams we can hover, walk through walls, do all the things that ghosts do. All our senses are active, but not in a physical way. When we dream, we are interacting (mostly subconsciously) with the astral world, where ghosts dwell. Very few people can maintain their sanity without these nightly visits to the realm of ghosts, which nourish our spirit and psyche in subtle ways, thus demonstrating how much more of a true home *that* world is to us than this physical plane.

For these reasons and others, we can say that you and I and everyone we see . . . are ghosts.

# Tips and Techniques

Before going on a ghost hunt, take a few minutes to do this exercise.

Wearing lose, non-restrictive clothing, go to an open room, stand upright, and close your eyes. Now, lift your arms out to your sides. Try to feel the energy that lies beneath the physical world, and within your limbs. Continuing to hold your arms out at your sides, rotate them in small circles with building tension. Feel how, through your will, you can increase your sense of the energy that forms your arms. Rest your arms again down at your sides, and for a time you will continue to feel that increased energy there.

Next, keeping your eyes closed, take a few steps forward, then a few steps backward. Feel the energy that is your astral body, moving your physical body.

Open your eyes.

Now you have a little sense of the energy world in which ghosts live; this may help you understand a little better the spirits you encounter on your ghost hunt.

(Ghosts are able to see, but their bodies are made of energy, even if they mistakenly suppose them to be still encased in matter.)

# Chapter Nine

## GHOSTS IN DREAMS

Sometimes spirits may visit us in our dreams, as we are then in touch with the astral world. It is easier at those times for ghosts to contact us—at night, when our conscious minds with their reasonable objections are at rest.

I once had a very clear dream of a friend who had recently passed away. He was a very close friend and my response to his passing may be of interest.

To backtrack a little, just before my friend's death someone else I knew died. For a while I allowed myself to fully experience the grief of that loss in my life, until a spiritual mentor offered another way to look at it.

"This is a very important time for his soul," he said, "during his transition from the physical plane to the astral world. If we care deeply for his benefit then we won't allow ourselves to indulge in grief and sorrow, which could act to bind his spirit to this earth. Instead, we should send his spirit on its way with as much light, love, and joy as we can muster, and a strong wish for his freedom from all attachments to this world. We should imagine ourselves in his situation, and consider what we would want to feel from our nearest and dearest. Let's send him what *he* needs, rather than thinking of ourselves."

I realized my mentor was right, and his advice came to mind when my close friend died soon after.

When I heard that my friend had passed away, I decided to forgo the usual grieving process—not through suppression, but by strongly focusing on sending him light and joy and a wish for his freedom in Spirit.

Every time he came to mind, I consciously sent him light. After a week or two it became a mental habit. A wonderful side effect of this practice was that just the thought of my friend brought me joy. When we wish joy to others, we find our own hearts soaring with happiness.

And now, decades later, I can honestly say that I have never grieved for my friend; nor have I felt a need to.

A few months after my friend's passing, I dreamed of him. I was in the middle of another type of dream: the kind where memories and subconscious thoughts are stimulated and blended.

I dreamed that I was granted the boon of three wishes. I came up with two wishes, which were instantly fulfilled. Before forming my last wish I tried to think of something important, so that it would not be wasted on a whim.

Suddenly, the thought entered my head, "Maybe I should wish for my close friend to be alive again."

As soon as I had that thought, my dream changed. It became less vague, clearer, more energized: less of a subconscious dream and more of a superconscious one.

I saw off in the distance my friend approaching in clouds of light. He had a radiant smile on his face. He was so full of joy that instead of walking, he was skipping like a child.

He stopped when he was standing right in front of me, beaming happily. Seeing him glowing with happiness, my impulse to help him seemed silly. Still, I asked my friend, "*Would* you come back, if you could?"

He shook his head, gazed at me with joy, and disappeared.

I woke soon after, conscious of having had a true visitation in my sleep. I have never forgotten this experience and what it taught me about how this physical world is much more empty and sorrowful than the higher realms of the astral plane.

This was a very positive dream experience, but other spirits can also intrude in our slumbers and those contacts can be unpleasant or even frightening.

I have spoken to people who have "woken up" while in the dream state to find themselves half-way between the conscious realm and subconscious sleep world. They became aware of malignant astral beings surrounding them and could hear their voices discussing them: an unsettling experience.

Happily, Paramhansa Yogananda taught a useful technique to protect oneself from such experiences.

# Tips and Techniques

Before going to sleep at night, slowly and very consciously write the sacred word "AUM" on your pillow three times with your right forefinger.

Alternatively, you can write the Sanskrit symbol for AUM (see illustration below). While you write this word, chant AUM* three times out loud with ever-deeper concentration. Feel that you are blessing, not only your pillow, but your bed, your room, and yourself with the pure and bright, crystal-clear light of Spirit.

This technique can also be used if one is afflicted with nightmares, to help ensure a good night's sleep.

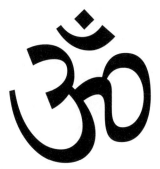

**The Sanskrit AUM symbol**

* To help you tune into the AUM vibration, I recommend *AUM: Mantra of Eternity,* available from Crystal Clarity Publishers, Nevada City, CA. Or you can purchase this mantra individually for download from iTunes™. Search for "AUM: Mantra of Eterntiy" by Swami Kriyananda.

# Chapter Ten

## HOW TO RELATE TO GHOSTS
## (A SUCCESS STORY)

I had an interesting ghostly encounter while writing *The Reincarnation of Abraham Lincoln*. I spent most of a month working at home, trying to kick the manuscript into higher gear, only to discover that the townhouse my wife and I had moved into was haunted.

Somehow, I seemed to have intuited we weren't alone in that place. One day, while standing in the kitchen, I clearly heard my wife walking down the steps from upstairs (*creak, creak, creak*), and the thought popped into my mind, "Wouldn't it be funny if I looked around the corner and Laura wasn't there?"

Smiling at my foolishness, I poked my head around the corner. My wife was nowhere to be seen.

As I started to pay closer attention to our experiences in that place, I became aware that, ever since we had moved into our new home, my wife and I had felt an atmosphere of emotional tension we had never known before.

"Laura," I said one day, "I think our home may be haunted." She agreed that we should have the place checked out.

By happy coincidence, someone adept at ghost clearing lived next door. We explained our concerns to Bill and he encouraged us to take a few precautions, such as hanging crucifixes on the wall and pouring a circle of salt on the floor around our bed at night.

He also made a brief reconnaissance of our townhouse and told us, smiling, "You have a problem." Bill said he had experienced an unnatural coldness in two rooms of our home: a chill he had come to recognize from long experience as emanating from spirits bound to this earth. Bill felt sure there were at least two ghosts in our townhouse.

Unfortunately, Bill had to go away for a few days. We made do in the interim but were glad when he returned and was ready to help our situation. He told us that dusk was a good time to explore for ghosts and asked us to leave our home unlocked so that he could enter and contact our spirit friends. We spent that evening away, and came home nervous and excited. What would we find? Had Bill been successful?

The first thing we saw took us aback. One of the crucifixes Bill had suggested we hang on the wall was now lying on the floor. What had happened?

Bill explained. He had started his investigation by entering our downstairs living room. Finding a "cold spot," he sat by himself in the dark. Before long, he became aware that a man was sitting cross-legged in front of him. He was a Native American and his face was covered with blood. The spirit was angry, and he said to Bill, "Death to the Cristos!"

Apparently, this Indian had belonged to one of California's Native American tribes between 1769 and 1833, when Spanish missionaries were active in the area. Somehow he had run afoul of the Franciscans, and possibly their accompanying soldiers. He had died with anger in his heart toward those who had killed him; and when the Indian ghost indicated that he didn't appreciate the crucifix we had hung on the wall, out of respect for his wishes Bill took it down.

(We also had photographs of our guru, Paramhansa Yogananda, on our walls; Bill said the ghosts were confused by these revered photos.)

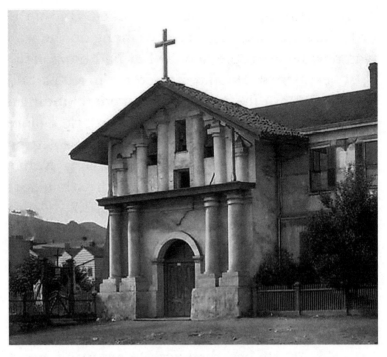

**"Mission Dolores," San Francisco, CA.**

At this point, Bill confessed, he was struck by a temptation. While in college, he had studied the traditions of the Plains Indians. Bill felt an urge to use the afterlife symbolism he had learned at university to help these spirits, but quickly dismissed that thought. No doubt these West Coast Indians had a completely different belief system, and so it proved to be. Bill drew out this Native American spirit, asking the Indian what he thought happens to people after death. By couching his conversation in terms familiar to the ghost he was able to convince him that he had passed away. In short order Bill ushered him to the other side.

Climbing the stairs, Bill entered the other room where he had felt another ghostly presence. Soon, he beheld a young Native American seated on a horse. This was the son of the man who had dwelt downstairs. He had been a very proud young man, and he had died with his father. Once again, Bill was successful in helping this spirit release his anger, acknowledge his death, and make the transition to the astral world. Afterward, according to Bill, the young man's horse dissolved into the floor.

When Laura and I returned after our evening away, the energy of our home felt completely different. It was as if there had been dark clouds in our rooms, but now bright sunlight shone through. Laura and I laughed joyfully and with relief while feeling the contrast—as stark as night and day. There was a feeling of freedom and joy in the air, where yesterday there had been tension and emotional turmoil.

Bill's actions on our behalf were deserving of praise and we will always be grateful to him. In addition, he had demonstrated a good example of how to tune into ghosts: how to be open to where they are coming from, how to listen to what they have to say—hanging his preconceptions, as it were, at the front door. But there was something else I wanted to share about this experience.

As mentioned earlier, I spent about a month in that condominium working on my book. Most of that time I was with those spirits and aware that they were there. In fact, there were many occasions when I felt their presence. My workstation was actually located in one of the rooms where Bill had said he had felt a ghostly "breath."

As you can imagine, this was an intriguing situation. Coming from the perspective of a long-time yogi, I reacted to it in several ways.

First, I practiced what I recommended earlier in this book: I watched my heart to see if I was becoming fearful. I knew these spirits could not hurt me, but (let's face it), ghosts can be creepy. Whenever I felt any fear, I stopped what I was doing and faced my fear head on. When it passed, I continued with my work.

In addition, whenever I felt a spirit's presence nearby I used a technique Yogananda taught for sending healing energy. I figured that those ghosts were in pain and in need of emotional healing. With that healing, perhaps they could detach themselves from that location and no longer be bound to it. Realizing their situation, I felt compassion for them and acted on it.

I also spoke to them aloud. "You are not in your physical bodies anymore," I told them. "Go into the light." I made these statements with as much heartfelt encouragement and goodwill as I could muster.

And so I passed many days with those ghosts, alone during the daytime in our house. In a sense, I got to know them fairly well. And I continued to bless them and send them light, to pray for their well-being.

Later, as I said, after Bill had cleared their energy and freed them from their emotional bondage and attachment, my wife and I reveled in the changed atmosphere. And I had an interesting experience.

I was lying on my bed to rest. Feeling drowsiness come over me, I entered a half-asleep/half-awake state, and saw two people hovering in the air above me. I forget their gender, but their nationality seemed to be a combination of Hispanic and Native American. They were wearing modern clothing, and they looked down on me with big smiles.

I felt these individuals were showering blessings on me, and wondered whom they might be.

The next day I mentioned this experience to Bill and asked for his feedback. Bill said that those spirits were probably descendants of the two formerly trapped Native American ghosts. He believed that they were thanking me for the good energy I had sent to their now-freed and departed ancestors.

I thought there could very well be truth in what Bill had to say. I felt at that time, and still feel now, that those spirits were my *friends*. If something really horrible had happened to me—who knows?—I might have found myself in a similar situation.

This ghostly experience had such a positive outcome that I recommend this approach to people who find themselves living in haunted houses: first of all, seek out someone who can free those souls, and in the meantime, send them as much light as you can.

# Tips and Techniques

***Sending Light to Departed Souls:*** The technique for sending healing energy mentioned in this story is a variation of the technique described in the chapter "How to Banish Spirits."

Sit in meditation for a few minutes. Then, rub the palms of your hands together until you feel the heat and energy there. Next, rub your arms to increase the energy flowing through them. Then, raise your hands and, chanting AUM out loud, send light and healing energy to any earthbound spirits in need.

You can also use this technique to send healing energy to your friends and family, or the world in general.

Be sure to keep your mind focused on your sending energy out, and not on the astral being who is the recipient, so that you don't create any unhealthy connections with that being, or allow them to attach themselves to your aura.

(If this is a concern, send the healing energy directly to the Infinite Spirit, and ask Spirit to pass that healing energy on to the intended recipient. You can also send the energy to your spiritual guide and ask him or her to pass it on.)

# Chapter Eleven

## GHOSTLY ODORS AND ASTRAL FRAGRANCES

In this chapter we will touch on a side topic connected with ghosts.

During the ghostly experience described in the previous chapter I can remember, along with other manifestations, a certain odor in our home when the ghosts were there.

It was a musty smell, but not very noticeable. Just barely there, and different from the odor one might experience from old clothing or wood.

In fact, I wonder whether it was a physical smell at all, or something I was aware of through the sensitivity one gains from years of meditation— something in other words not picked up through the olfactory nerves, but through the subtle astral ability to smell that lies behind the nose's function.

(Sri Yukteswar told Yogananda that "By sheer intuitional feeling, all astral beings see, hear, smell, taste, and touch." He went on to say that "Astral beings have all the outer sensory organs . . . but they employ the intuitional sense to experience sensations through any part of the body; they can see through the ear, or nose, or skin. . . . hear through the eyes or tongue . . . and so forth."*)

At any rate, I had a similar experience recently while driving into Virginia City to address a paranormal conference. The road I took carried me through a range of hills, and as I descended into Virginia City, I suddenly sensed ghostly presences around me.

(The feeling was so strong that, for all the time I was in Virginia City, I had the odd sense of being "underwater": immersed in the almost fluid-like nature of astral beings. Virginia City has been called "Nevada's most haunted town," and I would say there is good reason for that title. The spirits seemed to me for the most part benign, and I told conference participants that I expected Casper the Friendly Ghost would like Virginia City.)

Anyway, while descending from those hills into Virginia City, I "smelled" again a musty odor; this was a dramatic change, a sudden atmospheric shift while driving in a car with the windows shut.

I became curious about these ghostly odors and wondered whether others have had similar experiences. Since then I've done a bit of research

---

* *Autobiography of a Yogi*, p. 404.

and found that, historically, certain ghosts have been identified with particular odors.

It appears that there are various astral smells one may encounter, from the putrid to the delightful. And the stories related above were not the first time I'd had an astral olfactory experience. I would like to relate one such event that took place many years ago and was deeply inspiring.

At that time I was visiting friends in Sorrento, Italy. One of them decided to travel south to visit a well-known mystic, Natuzza, who lived in Calabria. Natuzza was a stigmatic (someone who bore, at times, the marks on her body of Christ crucified), and many people over the years went to her for spiritual help, advice, and inspiration.

My friend asked if I would like to ask Natuzza a question. In response, I handed him a photo of the Shroud of Turin. I requested that my friend give the photo to Natuzza and ask her whether it was truly the burial shroud of Jesus.

A few days later my friend returned. He described his visit to Natuzza: how it had gone and what she was like. He told me that he had given her my card and she had thanked him. He asked Natuzza my question and she replied that the Shroud of Turin was genuine. (The origins of the Shroud of Turin continue to be a matter of debate; for a number of reasons, I agree with Natuzza and believe it to be the burial shroud of Christ. My reasons are too involved to discuss here.)

At this point my friend looked at me curiously and smiled. He said something odd—to the effect that Natuzza may have sent me a second message in addition to what she had said.

I was confused and asked my friend to explain.

He told me that Natuzza sometimes sent a sweet fragrance, like the scent of roses, to people who communicated with her from afar.

I stared at my friend, astonished. "Ever since I woke up this morning," I told him, "I have noticed a sweet fragrance, like roses, in my room. I just assumed that someone in the house was wearing a new cologne!" The fragrance was very subtle, as if apprehended at the very edge of my sense of smell.

For the rest of that day I experienced that fragrance around me, along with a deep inspiration. And I remembered reading that Catholic saints like Padre Pio have manifested what has been called the "odor of sanctity."

Since that time I have noticed similar sweet fragrances unconnected to any physical sources like flowers or incense. They were always very subtle and represented moments of inspiration.

# Tips and Techniques

Through meditation, you will become aware of your growing connection with the astral world and how it can impact *all* of your senses: sight, hearing, smell, taste, and touch. Be alert for subtle astral manifestations and try to discern their causes.

Here is a meditation technique you can practice that will help you center and strengthen your inner consciousness and awaken your abilities to perceive astral manifestations.

Sit upright, in a cross-legged pose on a cushion (if that is comfortable for you), or on an armless chair, with your spine away from the back of the chair. If possible, face either east or north. Hold your palms upturned at the junction of the thighs and abdomen. Lift your eyes and, keeping them upturned, close your eyelids.

Keep your spine straight, but remain as relaxed as possible. Hold your chin parallel to the ground.

Breathe deeply for a time, in through the nose and out through the mouth. Feel that you are breathing in peace and joy, and exhaling out all tension and worries. Let it all go.

When you are ready, breathe in and out only through the nose, and watch the breath flowing in and out. Keep your attention on the breath and, as you breathe in, mentally say *Hong* (rhymes with song). As you breathe out, mentally say *Sau* (rhymes with law).

(*Hong Sau* is a powerful and ancient Sanskrit mantra. The words mean: "I am spirit.")

Say these words mentally only; do not move your lips or tongue.

Stay focused on the breath and the words; pull your mind back if it drifts away.

Practice this technique for a minimum of ten minutes.

After ten minutes (or however long you practice), take a deep breath, let it out, and forget your breathing, sitting quietly. Enjoy the deep calmness that comes as a result of this practice.

Try to incorporate this practice into your daily schedule. Speaking from my own experience—as well as that of many thousands who have done likewise—the rewards are well worth the effort.

# Chapter Twelve

## THEY DON'T KNOW THEY'RE DEAD: A FRIEND'S EXPERIENCE

You are probably aware that, like Patrick Swayze's character in the beginning of the movie *Ghost*, many (if not all) ghosts are unaware that they have left their bodies. Many of them think they are still physically alive, and are confused or even irritated that people can't see them or hear what they are saying.

My friend Raghu had a ghostly encounter while in the town of Warwick, England. He was visiting the cathedral there and, as a yogi, thought he would experience some of the church's spiritual vibrations in meditation.

Sitting in a pew located in a side chapel, Raghu closed his eyes. Immediately he became aware that there were spirits in the cathedral, including a man nearby and a woman kneeling before the altar. Although his eyes remained shut, Raghu was nonetheless able to see these ghosts, who were wearing post-Renaissance era clothing. Both the man and the woman wore the fine garb of the nobility.

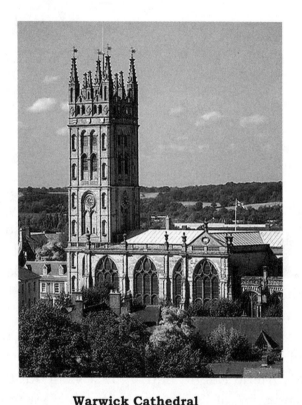

**Warwick Cathedral**
(Photo by Matthew Field; see: creativecommons.org/licenses/
by/2.5/deed.en)

As soon as Raghu noticed these spirits, they immediately became aware that he could see them. They turned to him with looks of surprise, and came to him. The woman arrived instantaneously. One moment she was before the altar, the next, she was standing in front of him.

Raghu said that he felt no fear, only a curiosity no doubt matched by what the ghosts felt toward him.

The ghosts seemed pleased that Raghu could see them. They spoke with each other and nodded in Raghu's direction, but he could not hear them. In spite of this, Raghu tried to communicate, speaking to them mentally. He sought to enlighten these spirits, informing them they were no longer in their physical bodies, even mentioning what year it was. Other ghosts approached— among them a dour-looking priest—and listened to what Raghu had to say. The ghosts' reactions to Raghu were amusing. They glanced at one another as if to say, "This guy is crazy!"

Raghu tried to encourage these spirits to make the transition to the other side, to go into the light, but he ended up leaving the church feeling only mildly hopeful that his words had had any effect. Perhaps they weren't ready to leave that place. If you go to Warwick Cathedral and are sensitive to such things, you may encounter those spirits there still.

# Tips and Techniques

If you would like to see spirits, practice the meditation technique in the previous chapter. Meditation makes one more aware of subtler realms. Through meditation, you will become more sensitive to the vibrations of places you visit. As I said earlier, meditation will awaken and enhance your innate ability to perceive astral sights, sounds, fragrances, and so forth.

# Chapter Thirteen

## GHOSTS AND KARMA

Paramhansa Yogananda had a number of fascinating encounters with ghosts. As a spiritual master, the astral plane was familiar territory to him. Once one achieves the highest Self-realization, one can manipulate at will the subtle laws that control the astral world.

At one point in his life, Yogananda's legs were paralyzed when he took on the negative karma of his disciples. He described the hideous shapes the lower astral entities were assuming as they attacked his legs: saws, corkscrews, and so on.

When one of the disciples commiserated with Yogananda on his condition, he replied, "It's not so bad. Other people have healthy legs, but can't walk all over." In other words, he was free to travel the astral plane at any time.

Yogananda also had the ability to free bound spirits.

One night when it was very late, Yogananda's disciples heard heavy clanking footsteps going down the hallway to Yogananda's room. The next morning they asked what had happened.

Yogananda explained that, in a past life, he had been a military leader in Spain. One of his knights had done something wrong and had accrued negative karma from his actions, which was still troubling him at the time of his visit to Yogananda.

The knight, who appeared in full armor, pleaded with Yogananda to free him from his bad karma. Sensing that the time was right, Yogananda granted his request.

But not all ghosts are ready to leave their bondage behind. Some are so obsessed with the past that they can't let go. Others, like that Spanish knight, have a strong karma which may bind them to a place for a particular length of time.

I gained a deeper understanding of this truth when I visited the Tower of London in 1993. Part of the tour took me through the White Tower—the original, central structure of the Tower complex that William the Conqueror had built back in the eleventh century. In the White Tower is a beautiful chapel dedicated to St. John the Evangelist. The chapel had been used by the Conqueror and his men for their devotions.

I felt inspired while standing at the roped-off entrance to the chapel. However, as I stood there, I also sensed very strongly and clearly the pres-

ence of ghosts hovering and flying about the cu-
pola of the chapel, no doubt drawn to this location over the centuries during the Tower of
London's bloody history.

At first I was puzzled.

I was aware that Yogananda had the power to
free spirits bound to the earth. And I also knew
that Yogananda had visited this same chapel
sixty years before I did. I was sure that he would
have known about the ghosts in and around that
chapel—in fact, their condition would have been
much more apparent to him than to me—yet he
hadn't freed them.

As I contemplated this question, I realized
anew that karma is an important teaching tool of
the universe. How can we learn our life lessons if
we don't experience the results of our desires and
actions? Some spirits may actually learn something from being bound to a location for a period
of time. Certainly, no spiritual master would free
them until the time was right to do so, until their
important lesson had been learned.

Feeling compassion for the ghosts who were
stuck in that location, I stood at the chapel entrance with my eyes closed and raised my hands
to send them light. (My actions must have startled my tour guide, who asked me if I was all
right.)

# Tips and Techniques

If you have the ability to help ghosts transition from the physical to the astral world, your work is a blessing to those spirits, as well as for anyone who may be tormented by their presence.

It is possible that every occasion of house clearing brought to your attention will coincide with that ghost's readiness to make the transition. However, keep in mind that each spirit has his own path to walk, his own karma to work through.

Try to hold onto a cosmic overview in your work, and if you find a spirit unready to make the transition, bless him, wish him freedom soon in the Light, and move on.

# Chapter Fourteen

## THE TRANSITION OF DEATH

What happens when we leave our bodies? Paramhansa Yogananda had some interesting things to say on the subject.

For most of us, death is something we fear, something we try not to think about.

Coupled with the fear of the unknown mentioned earlier in this book, the other great fear we face when we go ghost hunting is, of course, the fear of death itself.

The more we grow spiritually, however, the more the subject of death exerts a fascination. Why? Because some part of us doubts death's finality. In some deep place within we simply cannot accept that death is real.

When you have that thought, hold onto it, because it is nothing less than the truth.

In *The Reincarnation of Abraham Lincoln*, I spent an entire chapter chronicling a mental obsession visible in the lives of both Abraham Lincoln and Charles Lindbergh, an obsession with death that culminated in a belief in eternal life—a belief that would inevitably lead that soul to certainty.

Great yogis say that there is no such thing as death—or at least, not in the way most people think of it: the cessation of life.

The great spiritual master Ramakrishna said that the experience of death is nothing more than stepping from one room into another.

Swami Kriyananda, Yogananda's disciple, has stated emphatically many times that death is "*nothing.*"

There is no cessation of consciousness in the death experience; although some people may enter a sleep state when they transition to the astral world—either because their psyches need to heal from painful life experiences, or because they believe so strongly that death is the end of all life that their minds approximate nonexistence in dreamless sleep, or their awareness is not yet refined enough to grasp the subtlety of the astral universe.

However, for those of us who have reached a certain state of spiritual refinement, death is a transition to *greater life*. One feels *more* alive in the astral world, not less so. Colors and sounds and tastes and feelings are *more* vibrant in the astral plane. Those who depict in print or film a sort of hazy existence after death are projecting subconscious fears or expressing the lack of a refined consciousness. The only haziness that might come after leaving the physical body would originate in a person's inability to handle the intensity of the astral world.

In fact, knowing that death is a transition to greater life and beauty, great Hindu yogis and spiritual masters have traditionally celebrated their upcoming passing (known to them through clear spiritual vision) by hosting a joyful feast with their disciples.

This is the origin of Christ's last supper. Yogananda said that Jesus visited India during the eighteen "lost years" of Christ's life, unrecorded in the New Testament. Christ knew of this historical tradition and, fully aware of his impending passing (which he predicted), celebrated it with his apostles.

So, what happens when we leave our physical bodies in "death"?

Yogananda wrote that the first thing we experience is a sense of numbness throughout the body, similar to the numbness we feel when a foot falls asleep.

Next comes a very brief but intense feeling of suffocation. Simultaneously, a keen fear arises from the knowledge that we will not be able to use our lungs to breathe anymore. (This fear falls away as we become used to living in our astral bodies.)

Along with the feeling of suffocation, a lightning-fast review of our lives takes place.

Afterwards, our senses switch off one by one in this order: touch, taste, smell, sight, and finally hearing.

(Since hearing is the last sense to go, it is very important that we never say around someone who is dying that "there is no hope" or "he's gone." Sometimes a person will leave his physical body before his time, just because he becomes convinced from soyywwg he hears that it is his time to go, when it isn't.)

Then, Yogananda wrote that we may experience a deep state of sleep, much more enjoyable and restful than our normal sleep state.

Writing decades before books like *Life After Life*, that first chronicled the near-death experience, Yogananda explained that we then pass swiftly through what feels like a dark tunnel.

And then we find ourselves in the beautiful astral universe, filled with wondrous sights and sounds, and friends from this and former lifetimes.

# Tips and Techniques

For more information about the astral world and after-death experiences, I highly recommend the chapter "The Resurrection of Sri Yukteswar" in Paramhansa Yogananda's *Autobiography of a Yogi*, and the chapter "Death and Resurrection" in the book *Karma & Reincarnation*, also by Yogananda. Both books are available from Crystal Clarity Publishers.

Visit: www.CrystalClarity.com.

(By the way, the entire text of *Autobiography of a Yogi* is available to read on that same website.)

## Chapter Fifteen

## ARE YOU HAUNTED BY GHOSTS OR A PAST-LIFE MEMORY?

In 1993 I spent several weeks in southern England, mostly visiting historic sites. One day I traveled with a friend by train to the town of Battle and its ancient abbey, built where the famous Battle of Hastings had taken place nearly a thousand years ago (William the Conqueror defeated Harold of England there in 1066).

I hadn't seen my friend in years, and it was a pleasure to catch up on news and re-cement close ties. At one point we were walking in Battle on a sidewalk along an old stone wall. My friend was sharing a funny story and I was laughing. He was building up to a punch line . . .

All of a sudden, my laughter stopped.

Out of nowhere, a weight of emotional pain struck me so hard that I felt like keeling over. My mood shifted dramatically—a 180-degree swing. Moments before I had been in a light mood; now

I felt like that character in the *L'il Abner* cartoon who walked around with a rain cloud over his head.

I found myself short of breath. I could hardly speak.

My friend was still telling his funny story. Somehow, I managed to communicate my situation. Realizing the importance of finding the cause of these intense feelings, he kindly kept apart so that I could experience the battlefield on my own.

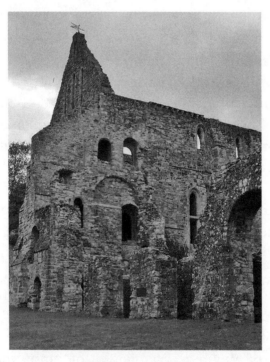

**Battle Abbey**
(Photo by Matthew O. Sloan)

If you go to Battle Abbey, there is a path that runs along the outskirts of the battlefield. Set up at different points along that walk are dioramas depicting what had happened at key moments during the conflict, which was over in a single day.

Audio headsets are also available that tell the story of that historic struggle.

I ignored all of that and walked out to the center of the battlefield, now a rural hillside that stands duty as a sheep pasture.

While sheep wandered around me, *baa*ing in the afternoon sun and nudging at my shoulders, I sat on that hillside and wept for about forty-five minutes.

I had an unusual experience then, unlike anything I've encountered before or since.

As I sat there, looking over the hillside and sheep pasture, I saw superimposed on that scene what I could only describe as a moving line drawing.

Soldiers hacked at each other with swords; horses reared; shields were raised; spears were thrown; arrows were flying.

I saw men dying before my eyes.

It was a very powerful experience—one I shall never forget.

The question arises: was this a haunting, or something else?

There are stories of people who, while walking on battlefields centuries after those conflicts, have heard the thunder of cannons, felt the earth shake with cavalry charges, and seen ghostly soldiers dying before their eyes.

Those unusual experiences filled those people with awe and fear, and afterwards they were certain that they had been visited by spirits—a haunting.

Certainly my experience bore similarities to what those other people encountered.

But, it wasn't a haunting.

Or, at least, not a haunting in the usual sense of the word—where one is visited by strange and unknown spirits.

I had been told by a psychic years before my visit to Battle Abbey that I had participated in the Battle of Hastings in 1066.

So the thought was in the back of my mind that I might experience a past-life memory there. However, in the moments before I had that experience I wasn't thinking about it at all.

The change in my mood happened instantaneously and without any forethought on my part. And the change was emotional, not mental.

It is possible for people to throw themselves into a mood by musing nonstop on a depressing thought. But I wasn't expecting a negative experience in that place.

When I visited England in 1993, I was aware of an interesting fact. The great spiritual master, Paramhansa Yogananda—whom many, including myself, believe was an avatar, or incarnation of Light—said that he was William the Conqueror (who fought at Hastings) in a past life.

So my expectation was that I would have an uplifting experience at Battle Abbey.

Another intriguing point: After I left Battle Abbey I compared current landmarks with old maps of the Battle area and came to a stark realization. My emotional shift had taken place just at the moment when my friend and I had stepped unknowing onto the old battlefield, hidden under the cement sidewalk.

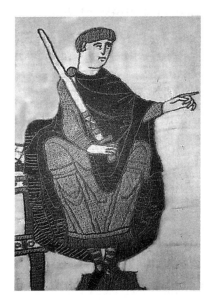

**William the Conqueror**
(Image from the Bayeux Tapestry)

# Tips and Techniques

Have you had a similar metaphysical moment at a historical landmark? One aspect of my Battle Abbey experience offers a critical clue as to whether your encounter was a haunting or a past-life memory.

While watching that moving line drawing superimposed on the Hastings battlefield, I had an *overwhelming awareness of personal involvement.*

The tears I shed were not for those poor soldiers dying before my eyes—but for myself.

In spite of the fact that, at Hastings 1n 1066, I had been fighting on behalf of a great spiritual leader, in that lifetime I died in a state of confusion.

My sorrow, experienced in 1993, originated somewhere deep in my heart and gut. I really felt as if I were letting go of something I had been holding onto for a thousand years.

(And, of course, if I'd truly fought in that battle, that would have been the case.)

I should say also that I have visited other historical locations, including other battlefields, and have sensed an echo of the pain and sorrow of the people who had died there.

My experience at Battle Abbey was *very* different.

If you have a powerful metaphysical experience at a historical location that you feel very deeply is all about *you*, that clarifies something deep within yourself, and that seems to be connected to something you are experiencing in life right now—chances are that it was a past-life memory.

A side note: I was reminded of my Battle Abbey experience a couple of years later when I saw Mel Gibson's movie *Braveheart*. You may recall that that film gave audiences one of the most realistic and graphic depictions of what medieval warfare was actually like. It really made you feel that you were there.

When I was watching those actor-soldiers hacking at each other, I had a visceral reaction. A strong emotion arose with me, and these words popped into my head: *"Oh no. Not again."*

In other words, I had experienced enough of that sort of fighting to last for all my future lifetimes.

I believe the Hastings battle was for me the last of a series of warrior lifetimes—and that much of my sorrow from Hastings came from my soul's recognition that I was ready to leave behind such violent altercations.

# Chapter Sixteen

## LINCOLN'S GHOST

My book mentioned earlier, *The Reincarnation of Abraham Lincoln,* is based on Paramhansa Yogananda's statement that Abraham Lincoln had been an advanced Himalayan yogi in a past life, and that he was reborn as the famous aviator, Charles Lindbergh.

*The Reincarnation of Abraham Lincoln* highlights nearly five hundred fascinating similarities and connections between Lincoln and Lindbergh—compelling historical evidence that reincarnation is true—and hundreds of connections between both men and the ancient spiritual science of yoga.

While discussing my book on radio shows, the question has arisen: If Lincoln reincarnated as Lindbergh (1902-1974), how is it that a number of people have seen Lincoln's ghost in the White House during the early to mid-twentieth century?

I have researched this subject. Most of the sightings apparently took place around the Lincoln Bedroom. One White House staff member was startled while opening the bedroom door to find the Civil War president standing there. Jacqueline Kennedy, too, said that she sensed the Great Emancipator's presence in the Lincoln Bedroom, and she sometimes went there to sit quietly and feel his inspiration.

How was it possible for Lincoln's spirit to be at least sometimes in the White House, and in Charles Lindbergh's body at the same time?

The answer lies in what Sri Yukteswar said about the various astral spheres. In the higher astral planes, spiritually advanced souls have a great deal of freedom of movement. In the lower spheres, deluded souls are much more limited.

Your soul is much greater than your physical body, or even your personality. Your inner spirit—more truly what you are than your body or personality—is vast and powerful. The more we manifest our higher and truer Selves, the more spiritual power flows through us and the more freedom we find from various limitations.

Swami Kriyananda, a direct disciple of Yogananda, once attended the Astral Ascension ceremony for a brother disciple. The deceased had had many good qualities, including a jovial sense of humor. But during the ceremony, Kriyananda was surprised to experience this man's spirit as so much more expansive and powerful than the lovable personality he had known.

Yogananda said that Abraham Lincoln had been an advanced Himalayan yogi in a past life. If this is true, then Lincoln's spirit would have fewer limitations than most of us who haven't yet traveled as far as he has on the spiritual journey.

Advanced souls sometimes leave remnants or echoes of their spirit in places, especially where important events in their lives had taken place. For instance, I have clearly felt the presence of St. Francis of Assisi in his favorite church, the tiny Porziuncula chapel, which he had helped rebuild and where he often worshipped.

More to the point, I've also experienced Abraham Lincoln's presence in some of the sites sacred to his memory: in Illinois at his home and law office in Springfield, and his old stomping grounds in New Salem; and his boyhood log cabin in Hodgenville, Kentucky.

Some of the most important events in Lincoln's life took place in the White House during the Civil War. That being so, it would actually be strange if there *weren't* Lincoln sightings in that historical building.

When an advanced soul leaves an echo of his spirit in a physical location, it is very different from your average person's ghost being stuck somewhere. There is a lighter quality to the manifestation—an orientation toward giving to others rather than needing help, a sharing with those who are open rather than a drawing within.

A spiritually developed individual can also be incarnated in a physical form while his or her spirit is connecting with people elsewhere on the planet. Just as some saints (Padre Pio and others) have been seen in two places at the same time (bilocation), the spirits of great souls are free to manifest wherever they are needed, without any diminishment of consciousness.

# Chapter Seventeen

## A "Lincoln Orb"

I am about the same height and weight as Abraham Lincoln and, after ten years spent researching my Lincoln book, I am deeply familiar with his history. Recently, therefore, I decided to offer Abraham Lincoln presentations dressing up as the Civil War president and talking about his life.

My first presentation took place during a Fourth of July celebration at Ananda Village in Nevada City, California. I stood in a tableau of former American presidents, told a few Lincoln stories, and recited the Gettysburg Address.

(You can view some of that performance online at: www.youtube.com/watch?v=xoTvALt8wEY)

The day before my presentation, my wife took some photos of me in my Lincoln outfit. They turned out pretty well, but I was surprised to see an orb floating roundabout my right-hand suit-coat pocket in one of the photos.

I found this interesting in that, while the photographs were taken, I was trying to act as an instrument of Lincoln's spirit—a spirit that had become familiar to me during my work on *The Reincarnation of Abraham Lincoln.*

Orbs in photographs are controversial. Some people believe these globes of light are manifestations of ghosts or spirits; others do not.

Whatever your own beliefs in this matter, I am publishing the above-mentioned photograph as something that may be of interest to you.

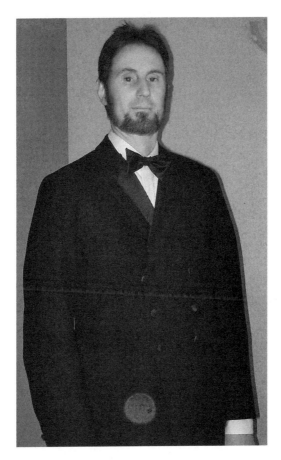

**The Author dressed like Lincoln, with orb**

# FURTHER REFLECTIONS: A FEW POINTS TO CONSIDER

I t has been said that if we could see all the astral beings in the physical world, they would blot out the sun. If this is true, the spirits we encounter on ghost hunts are just a tiny fraction of those we might connect with, even those passing through your room right now as you read this book. Happily, there is a veil preventing nearly all contact between the physical and astral worlds.

We should treat ghosts with respect. They are also souls, though perhaps stuck in a delusion and in a particular place for a period of time. Every soul is divine in origin and will eventually realize that truth. We should treat "stuck spirits" the way we ourselves would wish to be treated, if we were in their "shoes."

If, as a ghost hunter, you find that your mind and spirit become tired, or you are experiencing a period of emotional vulnerability, it would be wise to take a breather for a time. Ghost hunts exercise parts of your psyche that you don't often use. A ghost hunt is a high-energy pastime and it takes high energy to get the most out of it. When weariness sets in, you are less able to appreciate the experience. Better to rest a while and come back to it when you are refreshed.

I recommended earlier that you develop the quality of fearlessness. Another trait helpful for ghost hunters is non-violence (*ahimsa* in the Hindu scriptures). When we develop the habit of mental and physical harmlessness, of goodwill toward all life, the universe responds in kind. If you perfect non-violence in yourself, even if others on a ghost hunt are harassed by astral entities, you will remain untouched.

**A final note:** If you need help with clearing ghosts out of your house or your aura, there are people who advertise such services on the internet. I do not know of anyone who currently fulfills such needs ("Bill," who did a ghost clearing for my wife and I in chapter ten, is no longer active in that regard), nor do I do them myself.

If you have any questions about the yoga techniques I have described in this book, you can contact me at info [at] crystarpress [dot] com.

*I wish you safe*
*And illuminating ghost hunts!*

# ABOUT THE AUTHOR

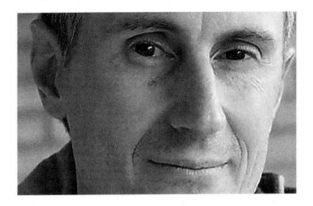

Richard Salva was born in Cleveland, Ohio. While in his teens, he became interested in yoga philosophy and meditation. He obtained his first job in order to visit a yoga community in Northern California called Ananda. (Ananda follows the teachings of Paramhansa Yogananda, author of the spiritual classic, *Autobiography of a Yogi.* Ananda was founded by Yogananda's direct disciple, Swami Kriyananda.) Two years later, Richard moved to Ananda Village. He has been a member of Ananda ever since, and incorporates thirty-eight years of meditation, and study and practice of the deeper teachings of yoga, into his writings.

Richard has written two other books—*The Reincarnation of Abraham Lincoln* (a critically acclaimed work based on a fascinating statement by Paramhansa Yogananda), and *Walking with William of Normandy.* (For more information on these titles, see the following pages.)

At present, Richard lives near Ananda Village in Nevada City, California, where he continues to write books based on Yogananda's teachings.

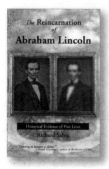

## THE REINCARNATION OF ABRAHAM LINCOLN
Historical Evidence of Past Lives
*Richard Salva*

Is it possible President Lincoln returned to America in the twentieth century . . . and we didn't recognize him? Based on the words of the great world teacher, Paramhansa Yogananda, *The Reincarnation of Abraham Lincoln* presents nearly five hundred fascinating similarities in the personalities, characters, and life circumstances of Abraham Lincoln and Charles Lindbergh.

The astonishing Lincoln-Lindbergh connections span every aspect of human expression and experience—from the physical to the mental, emotional, social, and spiritual. Parallel stories from the lives of both men demonstrate how the hidden laws of karma and reincarnation impact our daily lives.

**Praise for** *The Reincarnation of Abraham Lincoln*

"*****"
—FOREWORD CLARION REVIEWS

"*****"
—MIDWEST BOOK REVIEW

"A+!"
—DR. ROBERT HIERONIMUS, host of 21st Century Radio, author of *Founding Fathers, Secret Societies*

*"One unstoppable read of reincarnation."*
—SOMA B. DAS, Hinduism.about.com

*A compelling case study. . . . [goes] far beyond the realm of coincidence or superficial likeness."* —LIGHT OF CONSCIOUSNESS Magazine

### Accepted into the Abraham Lincoln Presidential Library

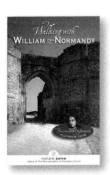

## WALKING WITH WILLIAM OF NORMANDY

*Richard Salva*

Paramhansa Yogananda told his disciples that in a past life he was William the Great (aka "the Conqueror"), the duke of Normandy and king of England.

Experience Yogananda's powerful presence and blessings in France!

This book is filled with facts and suggestions that will enrich your pilgrimage experience:

- Firsthand descriptions of the most inspiring William sites in Normandy

- Maps with William sites highlighted

- Brief history lessons to enhance your appreciation of each site

- Excerpts from the author's travel diary

- Photographs of William's castles, his tomb, his birthplace . . . and much more!

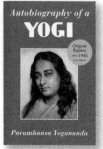

## Autobiography Of A Yogi
*Paramhansa Yogananda*

*Autobiography of a Yogi* is one of the best-selling Eastern philosophy titles of all time, with millions of copies sold, named one of the best and most influential books of the twentieth century. This highly prized reprinting of the original 1946 edition is the only one available free from textual changes made after Yogananda's death. Yogananda was the first yoga master of India whose mission was to live and teach in the West.

In this updated edition are bonus materials, including a last chapter that Yogananda wrote in 1951, without posthumous changes. This new edition also includes the eulogy that Yogananda wrote for Gandhi, and a new foreword and afterword by Swami Kriyananda, one of Yogananda's close, direct disciples

Also available in unabridged audiobook (MP3) format, read by Swami Kriyananda.

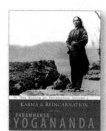

## Karma and Reincarnation
The Wisdom of Yogananda Series,
VOLUME 2, *Paramhansa Yogananda*

Yogananda reveals the truth behind karma, death, reincarnation, and the afterlife. With clarity and simplicity, he makes the mysterious understandable. Topics include: why we see a world of suffering and inequality; how to handle the challenges in our lives; what happens at death, and after death; and the purpose of reincarnation.

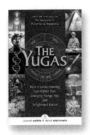

## The Yugas

*Joseph Selbie & David Steinmetz*

Given the tumultuous times in which we live, millions are wondering if we are due for a world-changing global shift, and what the future holds for mankind. Paramhansa Yogananda (author of the classic Autobiography of a Yogi) and his teacher, Swami Sri Yukteswar, offered key insights into this subject nearly a century ago.

They presented a fascinating explanation of the rising and falling eras that our planet cycles through every 24,000 years. According to their teachings, we have recently passed through the low ebb in that cycle and are moving forward to a higher age—an Energy Age that will revolutionize the world. They declared that we would live in a time of great social and spiritual change, and that much of what we believed to be fixed and true—our entire way of looking at the world – would ultimately be transformed and uplifted.

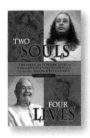

## Two Souls: Four Lives

The Lives and Former Lives of Paramhansa Yogananda and his disciple, Swami Kriyananda
*Catherine Kairavi*

This book explores an astonishing statement made by Paramhansa Yogananda, that he was the historical figure, William the Conqueror, in a previous incarnation.

The Norman Conquest of England was one of the pivotal moments in world history, a series of events that affects us even today. Is it possible that two of the greatest men of that era—William the Conqueror and his son, Henry I of England—have recently reincarnated as the great spiritual master Paramhansa Yogananda (author of the classic *Autobiography of a Yogi*) and his close disciple, Swami Kriyananda? If so, what are the subtle connections between the Norman Conquest and modern times?

## CRYSTAL CLARITY PUBLISHERS

Crystal Clarity Publishers offers additional resources to assist you in your spiritual journey, including many other books, a wide variety of inspirational and relaxation music composed by Swami Kriyananda, and yoga and meditation videos. To see a complete listing of our products, contact us for a print catalog or see our website: www.crystalclarity.com

Crystal Clarity Publishers
14618 Tyler Foote Rd., Nevada City, CA 95959
TOLL FREE: 800.424.1055 or 530.478.7600 / FAX: 530.478.7610
EMAIL: clarity@crystalclarity.com

## ANANDA WORLDWIDE

Ananda Sangha, a worldwide organization founded by Swami Kriyananda, offers spiritual support and resources based on the teachings of Paramhansa Yogananda. There are Ananda spiritual communities in Nevada City, Sacramento, Palo Alto, and Los Angeles, California; Seattle, Washington; Portland and Laurelwood, Oregon; as well as a retreat center and European community in Assisi, Italy, and communities near New Delhi and Pune, India. Ananda supports more than 140 meditation groups worldwide.

*For more information about Ananda Sangha communities or meditation groups near you, please call 530.478.7560 or visit www.ananda.org.*

## THE EXPANDING LIGHT

Ananda's guest retreat, The Expanding Light, offers a varied, year-round schedule of classes and workshops on yoga, meditation, and spiritual practice. You may also come for a relaxed personal renewal, participating in ongoing activities as much or as little as you wish. The beautiful serene mountain setting, supportive staff, and delicious vegetarian food provide an ideal environment for a truly meaningful, spiritual vacation.

*For more information, please call 800.346.5350
or visit www.expandinglight.org*